MALCOLM AYLWARD

How I Kicked Type 2 Diabetes Butt!

And You Can Too

Copyright: Malcolm Aylward
Published: March 2015
Publisher: Lone Wolf Press

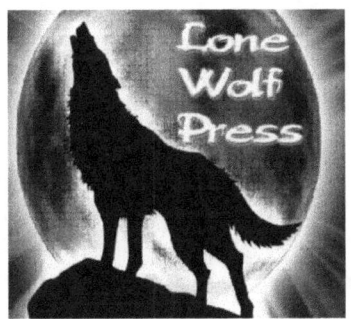

Table of Contents

Disclaimer

Before starting any new diet and exercise program please check with your doctor and clear any exercise and/or diet changes with them before beginning. The information in this book is merely the opinion of a layman individual. I am not a doctor or registered dietitian nor do I claim to have any formal medical background. I do not claim to cure any cause, condition or disease. The research and information covered in this book is open to public domain for discussion and in no way breaches or breaks the boundaries of the law in any state of the United States of America where I live. I am not liable, either expressly or in an implied manner, nor claim any responsibility for any emotional or physical problems that may occur directly or indirectly from reading this book. The opinions expressed in my books reflect my personal experiences and ongoing investigations into possible reversible conditions related to everyday health, exercise and nutrition.

Introduction

"My Story"

(True confessions of a former sugarholic)

Hi, my name is Malcolm Aylward and I am a sugarholic. Wait a minute—make that I *was* a sugarholic. Unfortunately, I have always loved chocolate and basically anything containing sugar and like so many of you, I have been wolfing down sugary pop, Twinkies, Ho-Ho's & Ding-Dongs since I was a small child, i.e. Augustus Gloop.

I was diagnosed with Type 2 diabetes back in 2004 and was forced to confront the sad and sobering realization that I was a full-blown sugar junkie. After much trial and tribulation I have decided to share with you my cathartic journey and explain in detail how I eventually eliminated the need to take diabetes medication and learned how to overcome and greatly minimize the harmful impact of Type 2 diabetes.

My goal and mission is to give hope, sound advice, as well as a simple and complete system that can work for anyone that has just been diagnosed with this widespread and growing disease. So if you are feeling lost, alone, confused, or overwhelmed right now I want you to please stop worrying. Just take a breath and let me show you the various methods that have worked very well for me personally in my ongoing fight against diabetes.

I will show you exactly how I accomplished this ambitious goal and, in the process, reduced my A1C and blood sugar levels to normal. I also managed to get my triglycerides, blood pressure, and cholesterol levels all down to normal range and got myself into the absolute best shape of my life. Just because obesity and diabetes are running rampant in today's society, that doesn't mean you have to board and ride that crazy train along with everyone else.

You need to understand the fact that there is no known cure for Type 1 or Type 2 diabetes. Anyone out there claiming they have a "cure" for it is essentially trying to sell you swampland. There is no cure. I wish there was, my friend. But instead of sitting around waiting for a cure, now is the time to get your butt in gear and beat this thing down.

There is no known cure for Type 1 or Type 2 diabetes.

I'm not going to bore you with all the details of what diabetes is and why Type 1 occurs because your pancreas can't produce any more insulin to regulate the glucose, or sugar in your body. And I know I don't need to tell you that Type 1 requires lifetime insulin injections. Or that having Type 2 means that your pancreas cannot produce enough insulin or produce it correctly to keep your blood sugar in check and you might need meds to regulate your blood sugar and control *insulin resistance*. Or that you could end up going blind with nerve damage starting to occur in your extremities if your blood sugar stays elevated for too long. All of this could very well happen, and more, if you don't start exercising, losing weight, and changing your lifestyle. Oh, crap—I just bored you didn't I?

Anyway, I'm sure your doctor explained all this to you and handed you many fascinating multi-colored pamphlets informing you all about Type 2 diabetes.

Luckily for you, I have already made all the dumb and painful mistakes that you won't have to make in your attempt to minimize the harmful effects of Type 2 diabetes. And that, my chocolate loving friends, will save you a lot of time, pain and effort.

Uncontrolled diabetes can lead to a multitude of serious health issues.

I need to tell you right now, truthfully, that your life and your quality of life are in great danger! Unchecked diabetes can lead to nerve damage, fatigue, blindness, loss of limbs and a host of other problems, not to mention— your untimely departure from this glorious planet!

Diabetes is extremely serious for it happens to be the 8th leading cause of death in the Unites States and around 285 million people are afflicted with it around the world. Type 2 is the most common being that 90% of those 285 million people have it. Nowadays more and more of our young people are being diagnosed with Type 2 because of all the garbage we feed them.

Diabetes is the 8th leading cause of death in the U.S.

Another scary statistic is that it is estimated that 37 percent of Americans aged 20 and older, that would be 86 million people, have prediabetes, also known as borderline diabetes.

Prediabetes is a condition where you have higher than normal glucose levels, but not high enough to be considered diabetic. According to the Centers for Disease Control (CDC), just 7 percent of those adults know that they are afflicted.

If your doctor informed you have prediabetes, you should count yourself lucky.

If your doctor informed you have prediabetes or if your blood sugar is between 100 and 125 then you are one of the lucky ones. If you follow the methods outlined in this book you are giving yourself the best chance to get your blood sugar back under 100 (normal range) and never have it develop into Type 1 or 2, if you keep working at it every day. Type 1 and 2 are not reversible, but prediabetes is thought to be. But you *must* take immediate and decisive action to lower your glucose level or it will most likely keep rising.

Here's more good news: According to a study in the *Journal of General Internal Medicine*, prediabetics who lost at least 10 percent of their body weight over a 6 month period reduced their risk of developing diabetes by 85 percent. Lucky ducks.

Let me take you down, because I'm going to…

Let me go back some years to the time shortly before I turned 42 years old. I went in for my annual physical and certainly was not expecting anything out of the ordinary. A few days later my lab results came back and revealed that my blood sugar had shot up to around 170! My doctor told me I had Type 2 diabetes.

If you get your blood sugar checked and it is 126 or above then you have Type 2 diabetes.

Needless to say, I was stupefied. I asked if they could kindly check it again just to make sure. It came back the same way. "Say it ain't so, Doc!" I can clearly recall walking out of his office feeling very shocked and dismayed, but also very determined to start eating better and exercising regularly. Or so I thought.

I went home and laid out my battle plan. I was to eat 5 or 6 small meals a day and go on a low sugar, low carb diet. I needed to keep my blood sugar as stable as I possibly could. I began walking and working out. Sounds great, right? I believe this lasted several weeks at best.

You need to keep your blood sugar as stable as possible during the day.

I soon fell off the confounded wagon and went back to eating like I used to and living a sedentary lifestyle. You see, Type 2 diabetes is a *silent* killer. You don't really notice any tangible effects from it—at first. But in time it will soon rear its ugly head.

Type 2 diabetes is a *silent* killer—at first.

I soon found myself lounging my free time away on the couch again wearing sweat pants while munching on Doritos, drinking Pepsi, and watching old *Andy Griffith* and *Emergency* reruns. Meanwhile, my pesky blood sugar was quickly creeping up and up and up. So was my pants size. At this time I was sporting a generous 38 inch waist and was literally tipping the scales at just below 250 pounds. Yikes.

After ignoring this most serious health problem, which the majority of people stupidly seem to do, I realized bad things started happening to my body. When I woke up in the morning, my legs and arms seemed very stiff and sore. My joints ached too. Periodically throughout the day, my hands and feet would just go numb and tingly. Sound familiar? If you are reading this book and have any of these afore mentioned symptoms then make an appointment with your doctor immediately if you haven't already.

My hands and feet would just go numb throughout the day.

I finally got out my blood sugar meter and tested myself one morning. It read 409. Remember, when I first went in to visit the doctor it was 170.

After ignoring the problem for almost a year it ballooned up to a very dangerous and ridiculous level.

The American Diabetes Association (ADA) recommends that you routinely test blood sugar levels as an effective part of your self-care program. I try to measure my blood sugar first thing in the morning before eating. Mine is typically in the 95-105 range every day, even with Type 2 diabetes!

At one time, my blood sugar was up to 409! Now my blood sugar is in the 95-105 range most every day.

I knew I had to do something, and quickly, so I made an appointment with a different doctor. Unfortunately my first doctor did not offer much meaningful help for me at all. My new doctor, however, immediately put me on a sugar reducing drug called *Metformin* and told me I needed to change my lifestyle or I would end up with all the complications of full blown insulin-taking diabetes.

That depressing news, combined with my feet and hands falling asleep all the time, spurred me into concerted and urgent action.

Find a competent doctor and work together with him to help you combat your Type 2 diabetes or prediabetes condition.

So read on dear friends and come with me on this magic carpet ride of what could be the most important journey of your life, to get your life back and to learn the various methods, including proper exercise, diet, & stress management, I personally used to wage my own private war and to finally:

Kick Type 2 Diabetes Butt!

Chapter 1

"Lifestyle"

(Cha-cha-cha-changes)

I would like to impress upon you a very important point. It is the fact that you have to come to your own realization and really make this a *lifestyle* change. You have to want this. You have to desire it and live it. If you can change your previous mindset then I can almost guarantee that you will get your life back and look and feel incredible. What I am saying is that there is hope, and you *can* do this. If I can do it, then you can definitely do it.

I have so much energy now, at 52 years young, it really is quite remarkable. My weight is down to 205 pounds and my waist is now a trim 32 inches. I practice martial arts, boxing, yoga and strength training and I love it! I go hiking, skiing, rock climbing, snorkeling, biking, and swimming every chance I get. I even play lead guitar in a local rock band on the weekends!

I try to eat as clean and healthy as I can and I don't smoke. I have cut way down on red meat, dairy, wheat & gluten. I truly am in the best shape of my life!

Since you are reading this book, I can safely assume that you, your child, or someone you care about was recently diagnosed with Type 2 diabetes or prediabetes. You have come to the right place. But if you or they don't become proactive right now, then you are putting yourself in jeopardy. If you do nothing, it will eventually make your life miserable and could lead to vision loss, amputation and other assorted horrors. If I sound harsh right now, it's because I mean to. You need to know the ramifications and the seriousness of this disease because I have felt the consequences and lived to tell about it.

You see, to keep your Type 2 under control, you have to keep eating right, exercising, and managing your weight for the rest of your natural-born life. You *have* to do these things to keep the monster at bay. If you stop at any time the monster *will* take over and your blood sugar will rise. A good analogy would be Tony Stark, a.k.a. Iron Man. He has to wear that magnetic device to keep the metal shrapnel in his chest from reaching his heart and killing him. Just like Tony, you have to exercise and eat right to keep your blood sugar from rising and possibly crippling or killing you. As long as Tony wears that device he gets to live. As long as you do what you need to do and control your blood sugar, you get to live too.

Fasting plasma glucose test. You won't eat for 8 hours before taking this blood test. The results are:

- Normal if your blood sugar is less than 100
- Prediabetes if your blood sugar is 100-125
- Diabetes if your blood sugar is 126 or higher

Hemoglobin A1C (or average blood sugar) test. This blood test shows your average blood sugar level for the past 3 to 4 months. Doctors can use it to diagnose prediabetes or diabetes or, if you already know you have diabetes, it helps show whether it's under control. The results are:

- Normal: 5.6% or less
- Prediabetes: 5.7 to 6.4%
- Diabetes: 6.5% or above

Depending on your A1C level (a test which allows doctors to examine glucose levels over a two to three month period) your doctor will either: prescribe you meds and recommend diet changes and exercise or just recommend the diet changes and exercise. I had to take the meds at first because my A1C was way too high. But as I started to exercise my A1C level gradually went down and eventually my doctor took me off the meds.

My A1C level is now at 5.5 which, according to chart above, is in the range of a normal person without diabetes at all. My doctor told me that it is the lowest he has personally seen in someone diagnosed with Type 2 diabetes. Before I became proactive and started my journey my hemoglobin A1C was 8.0, which was crazy high—off the darn chart high.

Before I started my epic quest, my A1C level was a whopping 8.0!

So you can plainly see that I have ostensibly reversed my Type 2 diabetes with this plan, but I have to always stay on the plan or it will most certainly not stay reversed.

Here are six *key points* that you can begin practicing right now, after you have visited your doctor of course.

If you are a smoker, you should quit immediately. Everyone knows that smoking is bad for you, but it is especially harmful to a person diagnosed with diabetes.

Point Number 1 – Quit smoking, because if you do smoke, you are:

- more likely to experience nerve damage and kidney disease
- three times more likely to die of cardiovascular-related complications than non-smokers with diabetes
- more likely to have problems maintaining proper blood sugar levels, because smoking raises blood sugar

Smoking not only reduces ones capacity to perform the work required to generate fat loss, it also directly prevents cellular growth and restricts oxygen and nutrient uptake.

Point Number 2 - Stop eating products that contain high amounts of sugar immediately and stay away from anything processed. Start eating foods from nature that have a low GI (glycemic index) like chicken, turkey, fish, fresh fruits, nuts, seeds and vegetables, things that are actually *grown* or raised and not made in a factory. GI is a number given to a food that indicates its effect on your blood sugar. This is not rocket science, so eat foods with a low GI. Feel free to Google any food to find its GI. Carbs turn right into sugar too, so you really have to monitor and limit your carb intake as well as your sugar.

Point Number 3 - If you like to put down the occasional 12 pack of beer or drink a bottle of wine, then you need to start severely limiting your alcohol intake from now on. I know, I know. It sucks. But alcohol is not going to help you lose weight and gain muscle. Alcohol is not your friend. So if you feel like eating or drinking something bad, then just ask yourself these two questions, "Is it going to help me lose weight?" Or, "Is it going to help me gain muscle?" If it isn't going to help you with either of them, then pass it by. You don't need it. You want a drink? Then drink water or green tea. Your will power needs to come into play now and stop you from making bad food choices. I will outline what my diet was, and is, in a later chapter.

Point Number 4 - Start walking in the morning if you can. After waking up, take a 45 minute walk on an empty stomach. Black coffee or tea is acceptable before the walk. Walking is a great way to start your busy day and get your metabolism fired up. I know it's hard, but this is what actors do to get in great shape for their next role. If you can't walk in the morning, then take a walk after dinner in the evening.

Point Number 5 - Get at least seven to nine hours of good sleep every night. Studies show people lacking sleep feel hungrier, make unwise food choices, and eat more (as much as 300 extra calories a day). Shoot for seven to nine hours of sleep per night, and try to get to bed earlier instead of sleeping in later. Good sleep is extremely important for your muscles and CNS (central nervous system) to recover properly.

***Point Number* 6** - Start your exercise plan today. I will outline the workouts that I did later on in this book.

In summary, please start following these 6 simple guidelines for reclaiming your life:

1. If you smoke, stop smoking immediately
2. Stop eating sugar and bad carbs, eat only whole foods with a low GI
3. Limit alcohol consumption, drink plenty of water
4. Start walking in the morning (45min on an empty stomach)
5. Sleep seven to nine hours a night
6. No matter your age, you need to start your exercise plan today!

Chapter 2

"My Journey"

(I'm Spartacus!)

By now I sincerely hope you are saying, "Pray tell us Malcolm; how in the heck *did* you beat this crazy Type 2 diabetes thing?"

Well, sit down, grab a chocolate protein shake and I will tell you how I did just that.

I would like to begin by telling you how the bizarre combination of gladiators, Bruce Lee, and yoga inspired me to change my life in so many amazing ways and helped me to practically eliminate my Type 2.

Flashback to 2010, a show about gladiators called *Spartacus* aired on television and of course, I had to watch it. Every guy and girl on the show was ripped and in incredible shape. When I looked up the show on the internet, I was led to the Men's Health *Spartacus* workout.

I noticed the actors that were in these shows all seemed to be able to get extremely ripped for their roles as ancient warriors. So I figured I would try to emulate what they did because, frankly, I have always wanted to look like a gladiator. Who doesn't? Supposedly the actors on *Spartacus* did this workout. There was even a video showing them doing it on the set.

Unlike most workouts out there, this one is not confusing at all and very easy to follow. This workout is a 60-10-15 circuit workout. That means you need to complete 10 exercises for 60 seconds each with 15 seconds of rest between each exercise. You rest two minutes after you complete one set of ten. Then you do two more circuits for a total of three. This is a grueling full body workout that you can do in 41 minutes. You will burn an average of 500 to 700 calories in that time and you will sweat—a lot.

The original *Spartacus* workout is free, readily available and remains one of the most popular and downloaded workouts on the internet. It is popular simply because it works, as I can attest to. You can find videos, docs, apps, pdf, etc. online. Pick a pair of dumbbells to start with that you can do 12-15 reps with. I started with 15's. When that becomes easy you can increase the amount of weight. If you can't complete the workout, then drop the weight.

Anyone can do this workout. If you have to stop and rest, then you stop and continue when you can. I went from a size 38 waist to a size 34 waist in just a few months doing this workout 3 times a week, every other day. As a result I am highly recommending that you to start the *Spartacus* workout or the workout of your choice today. I will describe the exercises used in this particular workout in a later chapter.

If you do the *Spartacus* workout correctly for three months, your waist will shrink and you will have to buy smaller clothes, just like I did. Just say NO to "loose-fit" and throw away those "fat jeans"!

Adriaaan!

I try to work in a cardio session on the days in between the *Spartacus* workout. I like to do a HIIT session or strap on the UFC gloves and hit the heavy bag or B.O.B. with boxing and MMA moves (tons of fun!). It is also a fantastic stress reliever. You can imagine whomever you like as you strike the target! Since I am not a big fan of running, I tend to lean towards boxing, the rowing machine, and jumping rope for my cardio. Boxers swear by the jump rope and they always look lean and hard.

The movie *300* came out in 2012 and also featured numerous ripped up actors. You can also find the 300 workout on the internet for free, but know dear friends that it is extremely difficult. Gerard Butler and crew supposedly did this very workout to get ripped for the movie. You can graduate to this one if you wish after you master the *Spartacus* workout. Be warned, it contains many, many pull-ups, which are very difficult for most people.

Row, Row, Row Your Boat

I read an interview with Gerard Butler and he mentioned he used the rowing machine to great effect. He said in the 3 weeks before the movie shot, he would jump on the rower and just kill it. That is how he got his abs to really pop.

You can get a rowing machine fairly cheap online, just read the reviews first. I purchased a simple one from a local store. When I combine 60 sec of rowing with 15 sec of rest, for 30 minutes, then jump rope for 600-800 jumps, I can burn up to 1000 calories in about an hour according to the Polar FT-7 heart rate monitor.

I highly recommend that you purchase a decent set of dumbbells, adjustable dumbbells are nice, but I prefer the hex ones. I do suggest getting a decent rowing machine if you can, a heart rate monitor, and jump rope.

The heart monitor is a great motivational tool in my opinion. When you can see what your heart rate is and how many calories you are burning it can increase your motivation.

The rowing machine is completely optional but if you dislike traditional cardio like I do, then give the rower a try. I will detail proper rowing technique later in the book.

The reason I shy away from traditional cardio like running is simple. Nothing against all you runners out there! But it really is murder on your joints. You only have so many miles on your joints. Once you use up all your miles, then it's all over. But if you love running, by all means, go run!

Can you say low impact cardio? For us slightly older folk high-impact cardio is not our friend. I have found numerous ways to perform low-impact cardio. Would you believe Yoga? (I will explain later).

You can burn an amazing amount of calories by hitting a heavy bag or a B.O.B. (body opponent bag) and have fun at the same time. I have slaved through endless miles on a treadmill. If you have too, then you know how boring it is, even with headphones and Van Halen cranked up.

Jumping rope is low impact and will burn calories very nicely also. Cycling is great but I really prefer the rowing machine. I always think of Gerard Butler "killing" it trying to get ripped for "300".

They Called Him Bruce!

I have always loved Martial Arts and Bruce Lee movies but as I rediscovered the new me I started reading and watching everything I possibly could about it. I took kickboxing self-defense classes and taught myself Muay Thai, Wing Chun, Jeet Kune Do, Shaolin Kung Fu, and Krav Maga. To my delight, I discovered that when practicing and learning these arts I was burning a tremendous amount of calories.

I have probably read every book ever written about Bruce Lee. I also have an extensive library of books about most all the Martial Arts systems practiced around the world. I also own many books on building muscle, nutrition, and exercising. My point being, READ! Read everything you can on what interests you. There is always more to learn. As the old adage says, "Knowledge is Power".

I purchased a heavy bag and eventually a Body Opponent Bag or B.O.B. made by Century. It is a male torso of a rough looking character on a durable mounting stand. The B.O.B. is extremely lifelike and made of a very hard rubber and can take a large amount of punishment.

You can practice all your strikes on the heavy bag or the body opponent bag. Knee strikes, elbows, head butts, jabs, crosses, uppercuts, hooks, combos or whatever you like. You will be sweating your tail off after about five minutes of this. I just can't say enough about this type of workout. Try a friend's heavy bag or a B.O.B. at the gym and see how it feels. I think you will find that it feels good and you will want one too. You can actually punch and kick your way to excellent health. What a concept!

You don't have to obsess over Martial Arts like I did in order to reap the many health benefits it can give you. It will work your whole body, core, improve your cardiovascular system, and make you stronger, not to mention it can lower your blood sugar and stress level considerably. I highly recommend that you give it a try.

Yoga, man!

I discovered yoga after a few years of lifting weights and noticing that my body didn't recover as fast as it did when I was twenty (DUH!). I tried some traditional yoga but found it a little confusing and complex. Not that there is anything wrong with that!

So I began researching other forms of Yoga and I was led to a style called *YRG*, or *Yoga for Regular Guys.* It has since been rebranded as *DDPYoga* after its creator, former pro wrestler Diamond Dallas Page. I know, I know—pro wrestling.

I investigated more and saw that Dallas had suffered a devastating back injury while wrestling. I guess those guys do get hurt, after all! While lying in bed recovering he noticed his wife had come upstairs after working out and she was sweating hard. He asked her what she was doing and she said yoga. Like most people he thought yoga was for girls. She convinced him to try it and he found that his back started feeling better almost immediately.

He then did his own research and came up with *YRG.* His back was healed from it and he felt better than ever. He had other injured pro wrestlers like Jake "The Snake" Roberts and others try it and it helped them too after years of abusing their bodies in the wrestling ring.

He helped many people transform their bodies with his brand of yoga. It really took off when a war veteran named Arthur, who had been on crutches for fifteen years, went from 300 pounds to 157 pounds and no crutches in eighteen months using only *DDPYoga. T*he video of his incredible transformation went viral on the web.

The well thought out 4-DVD set ($79.99, ddpyoga.com) features 11 distinctive workouts – ranging from a mellow 10-minute "Wake Up" routine to super-challenging "Strength Builder" and "Double Black Diamond".

I highly recommend *DDPYoga* to regain flexibility, burn calories, and generally make you feel fantastic. It helps me stay loose and limber so I can do my MMA and weight workouts without injury. I can perform the Warrior Three position for goodness sake. (That is the one where you stand on one foot, bent forward at the waist with one leg straight out behind you and your arms outstretched in front of you!)

I use a Polar FT-7 heart rate monitor while performing *DDPYoga* and I can tell you I sweat a lot and I can burn 500-600 calories in a one hour session. There are several different workouts on the DVDs. I particularly like the 25, 55, and 65 minute ones depending on how much time I have.

Big wheels keep on turnin'

I am not re-inventing the wheel here, for these are only my suggestions after extensive study and much trial and error finding what works best for me. Please remember to make adjustments as you see fit. You need to make it your own and find out what works best for you.

It's perfectly ok to swap exercises if you need to or change any element for that matter. Just make sure to keep it challenging, right? In fact I usually swap out the split squat in the original *Spartacus* workout for a different exercise like the burpee. The split squat is very hard on my knees, so I adjusted the workout to fit my needs, as will you.

Mental visualization is used by numerous athletes to achieve their goals. The great Arnold Schwarzenegger used to visual his biceps as boulders, or even mountains breaking up through the earth. Visualize how you want to look as you are working out. Accomplishing your goals will be 80% mental, 15% workout, and 5% pure guts and determination.

Diet is always going to be your toughest challenge, so please remember this: When something tempting and bad to eat or drink appears before you then chant this mantra over and over and over and….

"To achieve my long term goals I must sacrifice short term pleasure"

Now say it with an Ahnuld accent— oh yeah, that's much better.

Chapter 3

"On Cardio"

(On Dasher, On Dancer, On Prancer & Vixen)

I want you to look at a long distance runner's physique. Most of them are thin and not very muscular. Now look at a sprinter's physique. They are usually very muscular with great definition. Now I'm not knocking running, mind you, and if you love running that is perfectly fine. I have been there and I have jogged through the rain for miles and hours at a time. Did I get muscular? Not really, no. Did it help me lose weight? Yes it did. Was I losing muscle? YES!

Let's talk about interval and high-intensity training. After all the pain and suffering I have experienced, I can tell you HIIT cardio is *the* way to go. Doing short intense bursts of energy followed by moderate to light bursts is so much more efficient than traditional cardio. Your body will keep burning fat for far longer after a HIIT session than the traditional session. You can get more done in less time, and who wouldn't like that in our fast-paced world?

HIIT cardio is *the* way to go.

The popular belief that steady-state cardio is the best way to burn fat and lose weight is now being replaced by lifting weights and high-intensity interval training (HIIT), and the results are amazing. From Tabata-style workouts to weight training to sprint intervals, you need to be pushing yourself to burn off the stubborn fat that remains.

If you're looking for an excellent way to burn fat quicker and lose fat in the process, you really need to try HIIT. Not only will your body burn more calories *during* HIIT workouts but you will also continue to burn more calories and fat in the 24 hours *after* a HIIT workout.

If you think that lifting weights is the *only* thing you have to do to lose fat faster, you would be mistaken. You need a balance of weight training, diet, and cardio.

You simply have to do cardiovascular work to burn excess body fat. The body will burn primarily carbohydrates during the first twenty minutes of cardiovascular exercise. After about twenty minutes, the body switches gears and begins to burn stored body fat as the primary source of energy. You need a mix of weight training and cardio to get the fat to come off. Many people run every day and do not lift weights. Have you noticed their body shape does not change?

You have to do some form of cardiovascular work to burn excess body fat.

Sprinting uses fast twitch muscles, which take more energy to utilize, and it also puts you in an oxygen deficit or EPOC, so your body will have to play 'catch up' after the workout is done. This also increases your metabolism to accelerate more fat loss during and after the workout.

So after you have lifted weights, then you can either attack the treadmill or run outside. Or you can do your HIIT on the days in between lifting weights. If you are not a huge fan of running like me, you can also easily perform HIIT using a stationary bike, rowing machine, jumping jacks, jump rope, weights, even body weight moves.

Intervals of aerobic HIIT have been proven to increase VO2max (the volume of oxygen you can consume while exercising at your maximum capacity) compared to continuous aerobic training, even though HIIT workouts take less time to complete. A 2013 *Journal of Strength and Conditioning* study found that four weeks of HIIT rowing burned more body fat than traditional rowing. Effective HIIT training will help you burn calories, build muscle, lose fat, improve heart health, and increase your efficiency.

The beauty of HIIT is its ability to keep you burning fat long after your workout is over. You see, your body isn't able to bring in enough oxygen during periods of hard work. Therefore, you accumulate a "debt" of oxygen that must be repaid afterwards in order to get back to normal levels. The result: your metabolism is heightened for hours after. This amazing phenomenon is known as excess post-exercise oxygen consumption, or EPOC. The best way to use it to your advantage is to make short, intense exercise bouts a regular piece of your workout regimen.

Fountain of Youth

- For you guys out there, HIIT may actually increase testosterone levels. It can also boost GLUT4 concentration, which helps drive glucose into cells.
- HIIT also stimulates production of human growth hormone (HGH) by up to 450 percent during the 24 hours after you finish your HIIT session.

- HGH is not only responsible for increased caloric burn but can slow down the aging process. Can you say, "Fountain of Youth"?
- The American College of Sports Medicine has reported that two weeks of high-intensity intervals improves your aerobic capacity just as much as 6-8 weeks of treadmill jogging.

Please try one of these simple HIIT workouts below today and do it after your regular workout or on the days in between your weight sessions. Try it using a bike, rowing machine, jump rope, heavy bag, use your imagination!

HIIT Workout #1: **Power Intervals**

Go at maximum effort for 90 seconds, then go 50% for 30 seconds, keep alternating 8-10 times.

HIIT Workout #2: **Tabata-Style**

Each "set" is 30 seconds long, and consists of 20 seconds work alternated with 10 seconds rest. Repeat sets eight times for a total of four minutes. For the rest sets you stop moving completely, unlike the rest sets in other HIIT workouts, which are low-intensity but you continue moving.

HIIT Workout #3: **Turbo Training**

8 reps of weight training alternated with 1-2 minute high intensity cardio, for 45 minutes maximum.

Remember, these are just my humble suggestions that I have found to work very well for me. Feel free to modify them in any way that feels right for you and make them your own. Modify reps, weights, times, sets. It's all good.

Chapter 4

"Boxing, Martial Arts & Yoga"

(Punch, Kick & Zen)

According to stress.org, stress has been known to contribute to abdominal fat and other issues. I have found some interesting ways to reduce stress. By practicing Martial Arts, boxing and yoga I have reduced my stress levels considerably. Stress also diminishes your immune system, which we need to be working as best it can as we get older.

Question: What is one of the fastest and fun ways to ease your stress and work your abs and burn a ton of calories?

Answer: Throw a boatload of kicks and punches.

Boxing is a great way to lose weight fast. It's tough, engaging, and not boring. It is also an awesome abs workout. Your fists are hitting the bag, but your core is creating the explosive speed and power behind each and every punch.

It is also a great cardio workout. Boxing requires your whole body to be in synch so you'll fire your metabolism and increase your heart rate in the process.

Hugh Jackman, a.k.a. *Wolverine* uses swimming, running, and boxing to stay in amazing shape year round. Try it for yourself. If you have a heavy bag or a B.O.B., great, use it. If you don't, then you can shadow box.

Here is a great introductory routine:

Set a timer, (there are many apps for your phone you can download for this), for 10 one minute rounds, with fifteen seconds of rest between each. Each minute is spent doing one punch.

Left jab

Right jab

Left cross

Right cross

Left hook

Right hook

Left uppercut

Right uppercut

Jab and cross combos

Finally, go all out with all punches

Try to move around the bag as you are striking it, keeping your feet moving. Repeat one or two more times. I prefer to wear MMA style gloves, but feel free to wear regular boxing gloves if you like.

STANCE & FOOTWORK

Always keep your feet moving, shifting your weight from one foot to the other. The feet should be staggered and placed slightly wider than the hips. The weight distribution between both feet should be even. Both feet should be angled slightly to the side and the knees should be facing in the same direction of the feet. Having the feet and knees aligned will provide a more stable base. The rear heel should be raised with the weight placed on the ball of the foot. The elevated heel acts as the trigger for the majority of your striking arsenal and it allows your feet to be alert and move quickly. **Never stand flatfooted on both feet.**

Keep your chin down, your head tucked and your hands up in front of your face. Keep your elbows close to your sides and brace your core and always keep moving.

Here are some short instructions on how to execute the basic punches.

JAB
The jab is thrown with the lead hand. Begin with the knees slightly bent, feet staggered, chin down, and hands raised by the sides of your face (start from this basic fighting position before throwing any punch). Push off your back foot and snap the jab out quickly. The lead foot will slide forward slightly before impact. For maximum power, twist your arm in a corkscrew motion before landing.

CROSS
Also called the "straight right hand" (if you're right-handed), it starts from the face and follows an imaginary

straight line directly into the target. Drive and pivot from the rear foot, rotating the hips forcefully as your body weight shifts toward the front foot. Extend your right arm toward the target, snapping your wrist downward. On impact, the palm is down and the knuckles up.

HOOK

Shift your weight toward the rear leg as you rotate forcefully to that side and pivot inward on the ball of your front foot. At the same time, whip the lead arm toward the target in an L shape (the elbow should be bent about 90 degrees). Turn your hips into the punch. You can angle your hand one of two ways: vertically, so your palm faces you on impact, or horizontally, so the palm faces the floor (as shown).

UPPERCUT

Subtly shift your weight to the hip on the side of the rear leg. Dip that side's shoulder as you crouch down a bit. Next, with the palm up and the arm bent 90 degrees, forcefully rotate toward the side of your lead leg and push off the ball of your back foot, driving the punch upward (aim for the chin of your imaginary opponent). On impact, your palm should face your chest.

So, start with these basic boxing moves and gradually add in elbow strikes, knee strikes, and open-handed strikes, whatever you like. There are plenty of videos available online that demonstrate these moves. Wear your heart rate monitor and see how many calories you can burn. (Note: The heart rate monitor is not 100% accurate, but it should be fairly close)

Here is a Boxing/MMA hybrid workout that I currently do:

Left jab
Right jab
Left jab, right cross
Right jab, left cross
Left hook
Right hook
Left push kick
Right push kick
Left elbow strike
Right elbow strike

Left knee strike
Right knee strike
Left jab, right cross, left jab, right cross, left hook, right hook
Right jab, left cross, right jab, left cross, right hook, left hook
Left roundhouse kick
Right roundhouse kick
 Left side kick
Right side kick
Go all out with multiple attacks, move around the bag
Go all out with multiple attacks, move around the bag

As before, I go for 1 minute each round with 15 seconds rest in between. I normally go through both sequences twice.

Martial Law

I just can't say enough about Martial Arts and what a great workout it can give you. If you really want to have fun working out I suggest you take a local kickboxing class and see what you think. I would bet cash money you will be hooked. Most cities offer a variety of them. Check the web and be sure to read the reviews of the quality of the instruction at the *Dojo* or training facility. Unfortunately there are some that just want to take your money, but there are good ones out there too.

I had one good experience and one bad at two local facilities. I learned all I needed to from them and now I train on my own. Much in the spirit of the great Bruce Lee and his art, *Jeet Kune Do* or "Way of the Intercepting Fist", I try to find the elements of different Martial Arts that I think are useful and I discard the rest.

I own a veritable library of books on the subject. I also own several wall bags filled with rice for punching, the B.O.B., and a wallboard with a spring-loaded arm that I just love. It has a nice lower kicking pad for practicing low kicks. I hope to obtain a Wing-Chun dummy or *Mook Yan Jong* soon. Robert Downey Jr. is in great shape and happens to be a long time practitioner of Wing Chun and routinely trains on a wooden dummy.

Yoga Nights

Since I started practicing *YRG* or *DDPYoga*, my flexibility has increased tremendously. I have no problem doing the Warrior poses or some of the more difficult moves. This form of yoga amazingly can increase your heart rate to a nice level. When I first tried it and saw my heart rate go up just from standing still and tightening up all my muscles I could hardly believe it.

YRG uses a method called *dynamic resistance;* much like isometrics you create tension in your muscles as you do the movements. This added tension increases your heart rate. The dynamic pushups that you do are probably my favorite. And I do sweat doing these workouts—a lot. I try to do two to three *YRG* workouts a week. I believe it helps protect me from injury and stiffness.

Again, I am only giving you my suggestions as to what has worked well for me to reduce my A1C and blood sugar levels, not to mention my weight.

You surely don't have to run out and buy the *YRG* DVD's, but I believe you will enjoy them as much as I have. On my journey, I have discovered and learned to appreciate boxing, Martial Arts, and yoga as three of my go-to methods for keeping my Type 2 diabetes at bay. I am fully confident I will continue to practice all of these and lift weights for the rest of my life.

Chapter 5

"Weight Training"

(Lift to live!)

Weight training is one of the best ways I have found to reduce your blood sugar and control Type 2 and prediabetes.

When it comes to exercise, you have to train with weights to increase lean mass. Fat is burned inside of your muscle cells. The bigger and more plentiful your muscle cells, the bigger your fat-burning furnace. Adding muscle increases the size of the fat-burning machine hidden inside your body. Dieting incorrectly or exercising incorrectly hinders your fat-burning furnace.

The three rules of lifting you need to remember are:

1. Always use good form
2. Stay safe
3. Have fun with it

Work out at home or at the gym?

This is a question all of us face eventually. Some people love the atmosphere of the gym. I used to train in a gym, but because of time constraints mostly, I started working out at home. I also find the gym quite distracting and I really don't like waiting for a piece of exercise equipment. Not to mention the people who don't wipe their sweat off the equipment! I have quite a nice home gym set up in the garage and I can work out whenever is convenient for me.

When to work out?

Many people like to work out first thing in the morning and that is perfectly fine. I have to work for a living so it is hard for me to do it in the morning. The optimum time for me on the weekdays is right after I get home from work before I make supper. You need to figure out the best time for you and stick to it. Research does point to a possible increase in fat burning if you can work out in a fasted state, i.e. right after you wake up.

Things to avoid

Numero uno on my list is the treacherous kettlebell fad. These dangerous contraptions are causing more and more injuries all the time. If you use bad form you can seriously hurt yourself. I badly strained my rotator cuff doing kettlebell swings. The shoulders are not the most perfectly designed joints and are extremely very easy to damage. My form slipped one day as I was swinging the stupid thing, and it wrenched my left shoulder. It took over a year to heal and still causes me trouble sometimes. The only thing I would use a kettlebell for is goblet squats or possibly a doorstop!

Next would be machines at the gym like the Smith Machine, Pec Deck, Seated Hip-Abductor Machine, etc. These machines travel on a linear plane. Real movement involves movement in all three dimensions. So you are asking your muscles to follow the exact same path each time. Your muscles aren't going to receive as much stimulus from this range of movement and I believe more prone to injury because there is no variance. I would pick free weights over a machine any day.

I highly discourage you from doing Russian Twists. This cruel exercise twists your torso past the point where it would normally stop and can really cause some problems. I strained the connecting tissue between my ribs doing these and it put me out of commission for a few weeks.

Not being able to work out from an injury is not a pleasant time for me. I kick myself every time I do something stupid because it slows me down and hinders my good progress.

I prefer the hex shaped dumbbells, but you can use any kind you like. I also use an incline bench. I suggest wearing cross trainer shoes and not running or basketball shoes. This is my personal preference so feel free to try different shoes. Some guys love to lift in Converse Chuck Taylor All-Stars. Again, find out what works for you.

Start here!

I suggest you start with the *Spartacus* workout using dumbbells you can lift 15-20 times using good form. There is a link in the next chapter to download the pdf of the *Spartacus* workout for the exercise explanations. For men I would say to start with 15 pounders and women with 5 pounders. As soon as it feels too easy to you, then up the weight by 5 pounds. Remember to warm up and stretch before you begin any training session. I like to bang out 20 pushups, prisoner squats, and jumping jacks and do some groin, back and hamstring stretches before I begin.

Perform the *Spartacus* workout either 3 times a week with a day off in between or just do it every other day and take one day off to rest per week.

Perform your HIIT cardio session on the days in between the weight workout. If you can do it first thing in the morning, that's great. If not, do it when you get home from work or on your lunch break.

Here is what your typical week could look like:

Mon – *Spartacus* workout, 25 min of yoga

Tues – 45 min HIIT cardio w/ rowing, boxing, running, jump rope, etc.

Wed – *Spartacus* workout, 25 min of yoga

Thur – 45 min HIIT cardio w/ rowing, boxing, running, jump rope, etc.

Fri – *Spartacus* workout, 25 min of yoga

Sat – 45 min HIIT cardio w/ rowing, boxing, running, jump rope, etc.

Sun – Rest, take a walk

Do this for routine 3-4 months before switching things up.

If you like to follow a DVD when lifting weights then I would recommend *Body Beast* by Beachbody. It is an excellent strength program that features *Dynamic Set*

Training. The trainer, former Mr. Israel Sagi Kalev, knows his stuff very well.

Always practice good form, stay safe and have fun with it. Crank up your favorite tunes if you like. Lifting weights is a phenomenal way to get your blood sugar and weight down, so start the *Spartacus* workout in the next chapter and proceed to kick Type 2 diabetes butt!

Chapter 6

"The Workouts"

(We can work it out!)

Spartacus Workout

The *Spartacus* workout is one of the most popular and downloaded circuit-type workouts available today. Why? Because it works, that's why. This simple 60-15-10 routine can be done by anyone. So grab the free pdf of the workout online, then get an app or a timer, pick up your and dumbbells and let's get to it, shall we?

You will perform ten rounds of each exercise for 60 seconds before transitioning for 15 seconds and moving on to the next one. All of these exercises have videos demonstrating them on the web.

Exercise 1 – Goblet squat
Exercise 2 – Mountain climber
Exercise 3 – Single-Arm DB Swing (Alt – DB chop)
Exercise 4 – T pushup
Exercise 5 – Split jump (Alt – DB squat or burpees)
Exercise 6 – DB Row
Exercise 7 – DB side lunge and touch (Alt – Offset DB reverse lunge)
Exercise 8 – Pushup position row
Exercise 9 – DB lunge and rotate
Exercise 10 – DB push press or DB thrusters

Get the *Spartacus* circuit workout at:
http://www.menshealth.com/mhlists/high-intensity-circuit-routine/printer.php

Note that I switch exercises on three of the movements for various injury-prevention reasons. The three I substituted in are from the *Spartacus* 2.0 workout (which is also available for free at:
http://my.menshealth.com/workout/The-Spartacus-Workout-2.0/workout-a

You can try that one if you wish also or change them up every other month or so.

After performing the *Spartacus* workout for 3-4 months you should probably switch up your routine.

This next routine is one of my favorites as it can be done relatively quickly.

The Big Five

The science behind *The Big Five* is based on the five major movements of the human form. Pushing, pulling, hinging at the waist or hip, squatting, and the plank position.

This workout doesn't take too much time and many actors and celebrities are adopting it because of that reason. But don't be fooled, you still leave the gym feeling like you hit it hard.

Only do this style of workout no more than three or four times a week because it is a fairly taxing routine. Mix and match the moves and feel good about taking the less-time-consuming path.

Directions

Pick one move from each of these categories. Then do two sets of 12 reps. Change up the moves but repeat the plan three or four times a week. I usually do one warmup set with a lighter weight before the two work sets. Afterwards you should still have time to try the core moves and one of the cardio finishers listed below.

PUSH

Optimum: Bench Press
Lie face-up on a bench, holding a heavy barbell at your sternum, hands shoulder-width apart, elbows bent into sides. Extend arms, pushing bar directly above chest then pause and lower barbell to start.

Alternate moves: Push-up, dumbbell shoulder press, single-arm kettlebell press, push press

PULL

Optimum: Pull-up
Hang from a bar with palms facing away from you, arms straight, knees bent so feet don't touch floor. Bend elbows, pulling chest toward bar. Slowly lower yourself to start.

Alternate moves: Dumbbell row, TRX row, chin-up, cable row, lat pull-down

HIP-HINGE

Optimum: Deadlift
Place a heavy barbell on the floor in front of you. Push hips back as you bend forward, grabbing the bar with hands more than shoulder-width apart, palms facing body. Keep back straight as you stand up, lifting the bar and thrusting hips forward. Slowly lower bar to start.

Alternate moves: Kettlebell swing, Romanian deadlift, trap-bar deadlift

SQUAT

Optimum: Split Squat
Stand on your right leg, left foot resting on a bench or box behind you, and hold a heavy dumbbell in each hand. Bend your right knee, lowering until left knee hovers just above the ground. Straighten right leg, returning to start. Complete all the reps on one side before switching legs.

Alternate moves: Barbell squat, lunge, goblet squat, reverse lunge

PLANK

Optimum: Farmer's Walk
Stand up straight holding a heavy dumbbell in each hand, palms facing body. Maintain your posture as you walk 20 meters. Turn, repeat, returning to start.

Alternate moves: Plank, bird dog, side plank, suitcase carry

Extra: CORE

I also like to add one or two of favorite core movements afterwards. Following the same warmup/rep scheme as before, I like to perform the DB pass-through on each leg. Then I might add 30 ab-wheel rollouts or weighted crunches.

Or for those of you who have lower back pain then try this "no sit-ups required" ab workout and do as many as you can:

One arm DB suitcase carry

Pushup hold walkouts

Side planks

Fat-Burning Finishers

Throw in some cardio (and really fire up your metabolism) and add one of these five-minute bursts to your five-move session.

1) **Rep It Out**

Load a barbell with a weight that's about 70 percent of what you can lift one time, then choose one of the five movements and perform as many reps as you can -- without breaking form.

2) **Push It Real Good** – (My favorite)

On a rowing machine, row as many meters as possible in five minutes. Try to increase that distance by one percent on each subsequent workout.

3) Sprint-o-matic

Either find a hill or set a treadmill to a slight incline, about 3 percent. Run as fast as you can for 30 seconds, aiming for 10 miles per hour. Jog for 30 seconds at 5 mph. Repeat for 5 minutes.

Rowing

If you choose to get a rowing machine then please practice proper form.

1. *The Catch*: Sit with your legs bent and feet in the stirrups so your shins are almost 90 degrees to the floor. Fully extend your arms to grab the handle and lean your body forward so your shoulders come just in front of your hips. Keep your back flat and your core engaged.
2. *The Drive*: Maintain a straight back, tight core, and locked arms and then drive your legs back until they are just about straight. Once they are, hinge from your hips and lean your torso backward. As your torso reaches a 90-degree angle with the floor, begin to pull with your arms by bending at the elbows.
3. *The Finish*: Here your legs should be straight, your elbows bent, and you should pull the handle to your lower chest. Your arms should be slightly away from your ribcage, but not flared out to the sides. Maintain a strong core and a straight back.

4. *The Recovery*: This is a mirror image of the drive. The arms begin to straighten. When they are almost fully extended, the torso hinges forward from the hips. Maintaining a straight back and tight core, the knees begin to bend once the handle passes over them.

Always, always remember to:

- Practice good form
- Stay safe
- Have fun

In summary, feel free to try one of these routines or develop your own. The *Spartacus* workout is just my suggestion and I have found it to be a simple and fun routine that can take inches of your gut.

Some guys like to work one body part a day. Some like the split routine. I have tried them all and feel that the split methods are more for actual bodybuilders rather than regular Joes like you and me.

There is a huge amount of information and advice available on the internet and in books, some good, some not so good. I try to research what has actually worked for real people and see if it works for me. You will need to experiment and see what works best for you. I am merely pointing you in the right direction and giving you a starting point.

Now go lift!

Bonus: Arm Workout (Don't do this more than 2 times per week)

Using a fairly light dumbbell, bend your left arm at a 45 degree angle out in front of you and hold it steady as you perform 10 curls with your right arm. Then do 10 curls with your left arm with your right harm held the same way. After that, do 10 curls with both arms. Then bend at the waist with a flat back, bend your arms at the elbows and kickback the dumbbells until your arms are parallel to the floor for 10 reps. Repeat this sequence three times with minimal rest and your arms will be screaming!

Chapter 7

"Nutrition"

(Eat clean and prosper!)

My diet is fairly simple; here is what I try to follow all week:

Upon waking I drink 8-12 ounces of water. This kicks your metabolism into gear right away.

I might have a black coffee before I take a 45 minute brisk walk. After the walk I have a whey protein shake with 5 grams of creatine or one of my famous smoothies. On weekends, because I have more time, I might make 4 eggs scrambled with low-sodium turkey bacon and a small cup of fruit.

About 10 am I will have a half of cup of instant oatmeal with a half scoop of protein powder and fresh blueberries or Fage plain Greek yogurt with half a scoop of protein powder and granola with a little cinnamon (helps reduce blood sugar).

For lunch I would have a grilled chicken breast, one sweet potato (on weight training day only), and veggies.

For my afternoon snack I might have a few apple slices with natural peanut butter or a handful of almonds or a banana or other piece of fruit.

One whey protein shake right after my evening workout.

For supper I would have one grilled chicken breast or fish with veggies or leafy greens. I try to avoid carbs after 6pm.

That's it in a nutshell. I don't vary from this plan very often, so it makes shopping simple. The trick is to always have something with you or you will end up eating fast food. I never eat fast food and I advise you to do the same. Ask yourself that good old question: "Is this Big Mac and large fry going to help me gain muscle and lose weight?" I think not.

So preparing some food ahead of time is something you need to get used to. Just cook several chicken breasts on Sunday night and freeze them in Tupperware for the week ahead.

Former pro football player and actor Terry Crews stated that he always keeps a tub of whey protein in his car so he has something healthy to eat when nothing healthy is available. Hail Caesar, indeed.

Go Green

I think the *Nutribullet* is a very handy device for when you are pressed for time. This thing is a breeze to clean too. I might throw in some whey protein powder, creatine, veggies, frozen or fresh fruit, cinnamon, coconut oil or extra-virgin olive oil, natural peanut butter and water. Grind it all up and take it with you. I call them "Cancer Fightin' Smoothies".

Bananas are truly nature's power bar, before or after workout are optimum times for these bad boys.

Try not to drink your calories—stick to water, coffee, and tea. No more sugary pop or fruit drinks! And no Starbucks! Sorry. The key is eating as clean as you possibly can during the week and make good choices!

I always try to drink close to a gallon of water a day. People often don't make the connection that high water retention often means there's a lack of it in your diet. Not only is water great for you and your active, healthy body, but the alternatives like soda and alcohol are some of the very worst things you can ingest when trying to lose fat quickly.

Always keep healthy snacks around the house – almonds, walnuts, pecans, pumpkin seeds, baby carrots, etc. No, donuts are not healthy snacks.

When you shop please try to only purchase Low Glycemic Index Foods. You will have to do some research to find out these values. You can visit www.diabetes.org to find lots of valuable information on food.

You are not alone! Many famous people have revealed that they share the same illness that you and I have. Halle Berry, Drew Carey, Tom Hanks, Patti LaBelle all have Type 2 diabetes and are very active in fundraising and promoting awareness of the disease.

Go Paleo

According to Louis J. Aronne, M.D., Director of the Comprehensive Weight Control Program at New York Presbyterian Hospital/Weill Cornell Medical Center, in a recent article:

The healthy diet plan consists of the consumption of lean protein, healthy fats, and complex carbs. Foods containing Gluten, dairy products, alcohol, sugar, legumes, processed foods, and fatty foods are all forbidden foods by the Paleo plan. It incorporates nutrient dense foods such as sushi, natural yogurt, muesli, fresh berries, cereals, avocados, almonds, walnuts, fruit smoothie, grilled salmon etc. in five small meals of the day.

"Clinical trials have shown the Paleo diet is the best diet that can lower the risk of cardiovascular disease, blood pressure, markers of inflammation, help with weight loss, reduce acne, promote optimum health and athletic performance", said professor Loren Cordain, author of The Paleo Diet for Athletes and The Paleo Diet Cookbook.

Low-carb Paleo diet, an alcohol-free diet that emphasizes high-quality lean animal proteins like chicken, fish, and turkey, healthy fats, non-starchy vegetables, and excludes gluten, sugar, dairy, legumes, and processed foods.

I try to follow the Paleo plan as closely as possible. Both Joe Manganiello and Chris Pratt, amongst many other celebs, have stated they follow the Paleo program. Here again, I am following what seems to work well for these guys, who seem to be able to keep themselves in incredible shape.

Cortisol and Stress - The Enemy

Although many people don't know this, cortisol gets released from stress and a lack of sleep and factors prominently in body fat gain, leading to that pesky spare tire around the midsection. Cortisol raises blood sugar levels, which can cause fat gain. Cortisol shouldn't be feared, because it is a crucial anti-inflammatory—we just don't want too much of it.

Cruciferous vegetables are anti estrogenic, meaning they will fight against that hormone being active in your body resulting in fat storage. Increasing your veggie intake can help get you lean. Plus they're real good for you.

Now you know why your mama always told you to eat your veggies. Yeah, yeah, some aren't the tastiest, but you need them. Experiment with new recipes and spices to make them taste better and you'll be on your way to a healthy, fat-burning diet.

There's a reason that you always hear you should be eating five or six small meals a day rather than the three large meals that most people are accustomed to eating. It's all about managing cravings and to prevent overeating. When your body goes several hours without food, it starts to assume it's never going to get food again, upping the odds of eating binges and dangerous cravings. To combat that effect, it's smart to eat five or six small, well-timed meals a day to keep yourself full throughout the day and most importantly to keep your ever-lovin' blood sugar stable.

By the Numbers

I try to follow this simple rule: Eat for your target body weight. This is a system Alan Aragon came up with, a legend in the fitness industry. Let's say you weigh 220 pounds but would like to tip the scales at 180. You would adjust your calorie intake of a 180-pound man.

The formula: If you perform 1 hour or less of exercise a week, multiply your target body weight by 10. That's how many calories you should consume daily. However, if you work out more than that, add 1 to the multiplier for every additional hour you train. So if your target body weight is 180 pounds and you exercise for 3 hours a week, you'd multiply 180 by 12—giving you a target of 2,160 calories a day. You can divide those calories into however many meals you want—three, four, five, or six—as long as you don't eat beyond your daily limit.

Focusing on calories can work, yes. But by eating the right amounts of the right nutrients, you'll speed your results without feeling like you're on a diet.

Protein
Protein is the main ingredient for muscle growth. But it also helps extinguish your appetite and aids in fat loss.

The formula: Eat 1 gram for every pound of your target body weight. If you want to weigh 180 pounds, you'll eat 180 grams of protein. One gram of protein is about 4 calories. So to calculate the calories you'll be eating from protein, multiply the number of grams by 4. In this case, that's 720 calories.

Fat
For years, this nutrient was considered the enemy. However, recent studies clearly show that it's not fat that inflates your belly, but too many calories. As it turns out fat may actually keep you from overeating because it makes you feel full. The end result: You stop eating sooner and stay satisfied longer.

The formula: Eat half a gram for every pound of your target body weight. If your goal is to weigh 180 pounds, that'd be 90 grams. And since 1 gram of fat has about 9 calories, that's 810 calories from fat. This will be about 40 percent of your total calories.

Carbohydrates
Carb-containing foods not only taste good, but can also be rich in vitamins and minerals. So you don't need to eliminate them altogether; you just need to make sure you don't eat them in excess. And consuming the right amounts of protein and fat will make that goal far easier, since both keep hunger at bay. That's one key reason Aragon places a greater priority on protein and fat and leaves the remainder of your calories for carbs.

The formula: Add your calories from protein and fat, and subtract that total from your allotted daily calories. Using the 180-pound example, that leaves you with 630 calories. This is the amount of calories you can eat from carbs. As protein does, carbs provide about 4 calories per gram—so divide your carb calories by four to determine how many grams of carbs you can eat. In this case, it's about 158 grams.

You make the call – but be smart

Build your diet around whole foods—those you'd find in nature. I always try to buy organic and fresh. You should choose mainly lean protein sources like chicken, turkey, and fish. Make sure to include eggs, fruits, vegetables, nuts, seeds, et al. You can see that typical junk foods—

candy, baked goods, chips, and sugary drinks—are not on the list.

If you do happen to mess up and just have to have a piece of Grandma's Dutch Apple Pie, because if you didn't it would probably make her cry, then don't beat yourself up about it. Just get back to your routine and work harder. I hope you noticed there are no "cheat days" or "cheat meals" on this plan. You have diabetes, silly!

Chapter 8

"Supplements"

(What's whey got to do with it?)

There is so much information, bad and good, available out there on the matter of supplements. Believe me, I have tried them all and have come up with some recommendations.

Whey protein powder is number one on my list for many reasons. With the busy lives that we lead, it is very hard to get adequate protein during the day. We have to work, we have kids and commitments, and we have to work out!

It's really difficult to force feed yourself chicken all day, but I do try to take in 75-100% of protein equal to my bodyweight. Since I weigh 205, I would shoot for 150-205 grams of protein per day. You would have to eat six and a half chicken breasts a day to reach that! Whey protein powder is perfect to help you get close to your daily goal. You can find a list of the top ten protein powders at www.bodybuilding.com.

The two optimum times for whey I believe is first thing in the morning after your body has been fasting all night and within one hour after your weight-training session. I also use a scoop in a green smoothie drink or to make Greek yogurt taste better!

To be considered a superior whey protein the product MUST list whey protein isolate or hydrolyzed whey protein isolate as the very first ingredient. That's because whey protein isolates are the purest form of protein you can get, with some being more than 90% protein. And "hydrolyzed whey protein isolate" means that that high-quality whey has been pre-digested into smaller protein fragments for even faster digestion than regular whey isolate. Whey protein concentrate, on the other hand, goes through less filtering, which means fewer of the natural carbohydrates found in milk are removed. The result is a whey product that is much lower in protein content. So try to get whey protein isolate or hydrolyzed whey protein isolate if you can.

Creatine is next on my list. Information overload abounds on the internet on this subject too. I can tell you it definitely works, but—studies show that roughly fifteen percent of the population will not respond to creatine. You have to try it and see if you see an increase in size. Contrary to all the loading myths out there, taking 5 grams per day with a protein shake in the morning seems to work just fine. I always try to get *micronized* creatine.

Take your measurements before you begin taking creatine. I usually can see the most change in my biceps. After taking the five grams per day for a week or so, measure yourself again. If you see about a one inch increase, hurray! You are not one of the fifteen percent who are non-responders.

I have tried glutamine but I can't produce any evidence personally that it helps. There are numerous studies out there that claim it helps with muscle recovery. It is recommended to take 5 grams before and after your workout. You can find quality glutamine and other supplements at www.bodybuilding.com.

Branched Chain Amino Acids (BCAAs) are thought to be helpful for protein synthesis and for maintaining muscle mass while on a calorie-deficit diet. Other studies claim it helps with fat loss. I have tried them but I cannot see any evidence they help or not. BCAAs are usually taken right before and right after your weight workout.

Vitamin D is found to be deficient in many people. My doctor told me I was lacking Vitamin D. We need this vitamin for healthy and strong bones.

I have tried various pre-workout drinks and found they kind of make me feel weird, so I shy away from those. If I need a boost before a workout, caffeine always works, and it's cheap. And I don't mean Starbuck's! I mean black coffee, with no cream and no sugar or artificial sweetener.

A good multi-vitamin would be my last recommendation. But you need to make sure it is quality product. There are a lot of sub-par ones on the market being that the vitamin industry is unbelievably not subject to the FDA.

I have tried just about everything under the sun and these are just my humble suggestions only. One thing I definitely do suggest is to *always* keep some whey powder available in case you get hungry and feel like eating something bad. It is truly the *whey*, grasshopper.

Chapter 9

"Action Plan"

(Mission Possible)

Now I will outline all the key points and your "plan of action" to start you on the road to kicking Type 2 diabetes butt.

Consult your doctor before starting any new diet or exercise program.

Start here with the six guidelines from the first chapter:
1. If you smoke, stop smoking immediately
2. Stop eating sugar and bad carbs, eat only whole foods with a low GI
3. Limit alcohol consumption and drink plenty of water
4. Start walking in the morning (45min on an empty stomach)
5. Sleep seven to nine hours a night
6. No matter your age, you need to start your exercise plan today!

The Plan!
- Start doing the *Spartacus* workout or the workout of your choice at least three days a week every other day.

- Try a yoga session after the *Spartacus* workout (I highly recommend *DDPYoga*!) This will make you more flexible, lower your stress and help to prevent injuries. It is also low impact and burns calories.

- On your days in between your weight workout, perform HIIT cardio using boxing, rowing, running, swimming, jumping rope, etc.

- Prepare your food ahead of time. Make a shopping list and only buy whole foods. No pre-packaged crap! Don't forget to get a quality whey protein powder and always try to buy organic!

- Try the Paleo Diet or a modified version of it.

- Never, ever, ever eat fast food. It's poison.

- Drink plenty of H2O! Keep hydrated at all times.

- Get out in nature and take walks or hikes often because we need the sunshine for serotonin and Vitamin D, which helps us fight off depression, provide protection against colds, and a host of other benefits.

- Monitor your blood sugar every day and communicate with your doctor about any drastic changes.

- Take at least one day a week as a rest day or just take a short walk. Your central nervous system needs some time to recover.

- Never stop learning, read all you can, study, and experiment. This is all about you, so keep it safe and make it your own!

Recommended Gear
Blood sugar meter
Heart rate monitor (optional)
Jump rope
Rowing machine (optional)
Incline weight bench
Dumbbells and/or weights
Ab Roller
Heavy bag or B.O.B.
Boxing or MMA gloves
Cross trainer shoes

Chapter 10

"Closing Thoughts"

(Na-na na na, hey hey hey, goodbye)

I hope you have enjoyed this book as much as I did writing it. I take great pride in the fact that I, for all intents and purposes, have kicked Type 2's royal butt!

Not only is it generally a good idea to get checked out by your doctor on a regular basis, but it's also essential if you want to make sure your body is in peak physical condition for hitting the gym, running, or doing any kind of fitness regimen.

It's especially important to have your thyroid checked to make sure you're not suffering from hypothyroidism (or, in layman's terms, an underactive thyroid gland). You see the thyroid gland controls your body's metabolism. With that in mind, it's essential to ensure that your thyroid is working correctly if you want to lose weight (or avoid possible weight *gain*). If you're having trouble losing weight (and you're staying active and eating right), you might need to get that thyroid checked out.

I would suggest taking photos before, after, and during your journey because it is a *great* way to stay motivated throughout the entire sweat-inducing ordeal. You will get to *see* the fruits of your labor as your stomach flattens, your skin tightens up, your face thins out, and your body transforms into a lean, mean, fat-burning machine.

Picking up a sport (especially getting into pick-up games) is a great way to burn extra calories, trim away the fat and still have a lot of fun doing it. Go shoot some hoops with the kids!

Playing a sport involves cardio and lots of non-linear movement (jumping, back pedaling, side stepping) making it healthier than straight jogging. Plus it keeps you having fun without getting too bored.

You can walk into any gym in America and you can watch the gym rats performing the exact same workout three times per week. They all do cardio for 30-60 minutes followed by a trip around the weight room. You need to change it up periodically. 30 minutes of high intensity lifting followed by 15 minutes of high intensity intervals will produce more results in two days than your standard 90-minute workout three days a week.

Are you a scale-watcher? Do you step on the scale every morning before you get dressed? Well, cut it out already! If you've been going to the gym every day, eating right, and staying active there's a good chance you don't see your weight go down because, as you're losing fat, you're also gaining muscle. Muscle weighs more than fat. Remember to not depend on the scale. Weigh yourself once or twice a week and use your tape measure instead of the scale to track your progress. I strongly feel that the best indicator of progress is looking in the mirror and to simply ask oneself, "How do my clothes fit?"

Get off your butt and move! Start taking the stairs, and not the elevator. There are many ways to reprogram your brain and start burning away the fat: Switch to a standing (or treadmill) desk. Knock out a set of pushups or jumping jacks during the commercials when you're watching TV. Get the picture? Just get up and keep moving.

Walk more and drive less. The more you walk, the more active you are. The more active you are, the more calories you burn, and the more weight you can potentially lose. Instead of driving up the street to grab your java, take a nice walk up and back. If you want to take the family to the park for an hour, leave the car and hit the pavement instead. Not only will you save money on gas, but also you and your family will benefit greatly from it.

Lacking proper sleep is a surefire way to gain weight. When you are sleep deprived your body reacts in different ways on a hormonal level, which can hinder weight loss. During times of sleep deprivation your body is on high alert thinking that there is a danger (or else you would be sleeping), so your metabolism slows way down to conserve energy. Second, your appetite is higher (due to elevated levels of cortisol) looking for food for more energy. Third, your food choices becomes affected in that your body tends to crave high carbohydrate, high fat foods because they help produce serotonin, which helps calm you down from this state.

Find a workout partner! I do prefer to work out alone, but having a workout buddy is also a great idea. It's all about motivation. You pull each other out of the blues and into the world of health and fitness. Just when you think you can't run any farther or do that last rep, you have your buddy there to make *sure* you do it.

Crank up the tunes! Studies have shown that listening to motivating music while working out can increase intensity which translates to better gains for you in the time spent.

One of the most important ways to ensure that you continue to eat healthy is to be aware of everything that you put into your body. And what better way to do that than with some of the apps made for the device you always have with you – your phone! There are tons of applications made for iPhone, iPad, Android, Mac and PCs. Not only do they provide great visual and quantitative feedback about the calories you're ingesting, but it's also a good way to take a step back, breath, and really think about what you're putting in your body at every meal.

In closing, I would like to thank you personally for taking the time to read this book and share in my journey. I hope I have ignited that spark in you by showing that you can truly beat this thing. You *can* slay the Type 2 diabetes dragon using the methods that I have outlined for you here.

I always like to look for and recognize the positive in people, in the world, and in life. Even though it totally sucked when I found out I did indeed have Type 2, I can see the positive in it now. If it weren't for Type 2 diabetes, I might not have reduced my weight and gotten myself in the great shape that I am in today. I could have developed high blood pressure, high cholesterol, clogged arteries, or any number of things that could have sidelined me if I hadn't taken action.

So, my friend, I wholeheartedly urge you to begin this epic journey today. There is not a moment to lose. Your quality of life, your health and your loved ones are all depending on you and the smart choices you need to make. Take back your life and start living again, stay focused, stay safe, be positive and know that using these proven methods, you can most definitely:

KICK TYPE 2 DIABETES BUTT!

Please feel free to leave a review on Amazon.com

amazon.com/author/malcolmaylward

Veni, Vedi, Vici!
(I came, I saw, I conquered!)

Great web sites with good information:
Diabetes.org
Menshealth.com
Mensfitness.com
Health.com/health/celebrity-tips.com
Bodybuilding.com

How I Kicked Type 2 Diabetes Butt!

And You Can Too

Published by

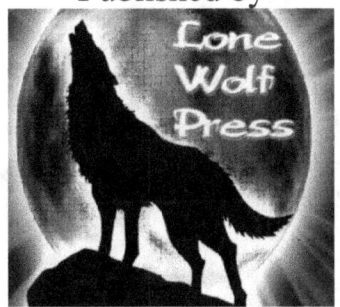

Lone Wolf Press

MALCOLM AYLWARD

Web Site - malcolmaylwardbooks.com
Twitter - twitter.com/malcolmaylward
Facebook - facebook.com/malcolmaylwardbooks
Blog - malcolmaylwardbooks.com.blogspot.com
Mailing List - malcolmaylwardbooks.com/mailing-list.html